NUTRITION AND DIET THERAPY

A Comprehensive Guide to Optimal Health and Wellness

DR. RAYMOND F. BERNARD

Copyright © [2023] by [Dr. Raymond F. Bernard]

All rights reserved.

No part of this publication may be reproduced,
Distributed, or transmitted in any form or by any means, including photocopying, recording, or other electronic or Mechanical methods, Without the prior written Permission of the publisher Except in the case of brief quotations embodied in critical reviews and certain other

Publish by Dr. Raymond F. Bernard

Disclaimer: the opinion and views expressed in this book are those of the author and do not necessarily reflect the policy or position of any character or organization mention in this book

TABLE OF CONTENTS

CHAPTER 1

Introduction to Nutrition and Diet Therapy

In this opening chapter of our journey into the world of nutrition and diet therapy, we lay the foundation for understanding why what we eat matters so much for our health and well-being. It's like the prologue of a book, setting the stage for the critical topics we'll delve into throughout the rest of our exploration.

Why Nutrition Matters: A Vital Introduction

At its core, nutrition is about the food we eat and how it affects our bodies. Every meal you consume is essentially a package of nutrients, and these nutrients have a profound impact on your health. Imagine your body as a finely tuned machine, and the fuel for this machine is the food you consume. Just as a car requires the right type of fuel to run efficiently, your body relies on the right balance of nutrients to function optimally.

Nutrition isn't just about avoiding hunger; it's about providing your body with the essential elements it needs to thrive. These elements include macronutrients like carbohydrates, proteins, and fats, as well as micronutrients like vitamins and minerals. We'll dive into these nutrients in more detail in later chapters, but for now, it's crucial to understand that each plays a unique role in your overall health.

Historical Perspective on Diet Therapy

To truly appreciate the significance of nutrition, we need to briefly journey through its historical evolution. People have recognized the link between food and health for millennia, although our understanding has deepened over time.

Throughout history, various cultures and civilizations have employed diet as a form of therapy. Ancient Greeks, for instance, believed in the healing properties of specific foods and diets. Hippocrates, often regarded as the father of medicine, famously said, "Let food be thy medicine, and medicine be thy food." This wisdom laid the early foundation for what we now call diet therapy.

In more recent history, the role of diet in preventing and managing diseases became increasingly evident. The discovery of essential vitamins and minerals in the early 20th century marked a significant turning point in our understanding of nutrition's role in health.

Fast forward to today, and we have a wealth of scientific knowledge about how different nutrients impact our bodies. We've come a long way from ancient beliefs and are now armed with data-backed insights into the complex relationship between diet and health.

Key Terms and Concepts in Nutrition

Like any field, nutrition has its own language and terminology. Let's break down some key terms and concepts that will be recurring themes throughout this book:

1. **Nutrients:** These are the chemical compounds found in food that nourish your body. Nutrients can be classified into two main categories: macronutrients and micronutrients.

   - **Macronutrients:** These are the nutrients your body needs in larger quantities. They include carbohydrates (which provide energy), proteins (essential for growth and repair), and fats (important for energy storage and cell structure).

- **Micronutrients:** These are nutrients required in smaller quantities but are equally vital. Vitamins and minerals fall into this category, and they play crucial roles in various bodily functions.

2. **Calories:** You've likely heard this term before. Calories are units of energy derived from the food you eat. Your body needs a certain number of calories to maintain its functions, and consuming too many or too few can lead to weight gain or loss.

3. **Metabolism:** This term refers to all the chemical processes that occur within your body to maintain life. Your metabolism dictates how quickly you burn

calories and how efficiently your body utilizes nutrients.

4. **Recommended Dietary Allowances (RDAs):** These are guidelines set by health authorities to inform individuals about the daily intake of various nutrients needed to maintain good health. RDAs are often used as reference points to evaluate the adequacy of one's diet.

5. **Dietitian vs. Nutritionist:** You might have heard these terms used interchangeably, but they have distinct differences.

Dietitians typically have formal education and training in dietetics, including clinical nutrition and therapeutic diets. They often work in clinical settings. Nutritionists, on the other hand, can have various levels of training and may focus more on general nutrition and wellness.

6. **Balanced Diet:** This is a fundamental concept. A balanced diet means getting the right amount of nutrients from a variety of foods to support overall health. It's like a nutritional

jigsaw puzzle where each piece (food group) is essential for the complete picture of well-being.

The Role of Dietitians and Nutritionists

As we delve deeper into the world of nutrition and diet therapy, it's essential to understand the professionals who play a crucial role in guiding individuals and communities toward healthier eating habits.

Dietitians are experts in food and nutrition. They typically hold degrees in dietetics, nutrition, or a related field, and many are registered dietitians (RDs) or registered dietitian nutritionists (RDNs). This registration involves meeting specific educational and professional requirements and passing a national exam.

Dietitians work in various settings, including hospitals, clinics, schools, and public health agencies. They provide personalized nutrition advice, develop dietary plans for individuals with specific medical conditions, and often collaborate with healthcare teams to ensure patients receive appropriate nutrition during illness and recovery.

Nutritionists also focus on nutrition but may have varying levels of formal education and training. The term "nutritionist" isn't regulated in the same way as "dietitian," which means that individuals with different backgrounds and qualifications can use it. Some nutritionists may offer general dietary advice and support for wellness, while others may have specialized knowledge in certain areas of nutrition.

In practical terms, whether you seek advice from a dietitian or nutritionist depends on your specific needs. If you have a medical condition, such as diabetes or heart disease, or if you're seeking personalized dietary guidance, consulting a registered dietitian is often recommended. For general nutrition advice and wellness goals, a nutritionist may suffice.

As we move forward in this book, you'll gain a deeper appreciation for the role of these professionals in helping individuals and communities make informed choices about their diets. Additionally, you'll discover how understanding nutrition can empower you to take control of your health and well-being.

In conclusion, Chapter 1 serves as the opening act of our exploration into the fascinating world of nutrition and diet therapy. It lays the groundwork by emphasizing the crucial role nutrition plays in our lives and briefly delves into its historical context. We've also introduced key terms and concepts that will become second nature as we progress through the chapters. Lastly, we've touched on the roles of dietitians and nutritionists, who will be our guides on this journey toward better health through informed eating.

CHAPTER 2

Macronutrients - Carbohydrates, Proteins, and Fats

Welcome to Chapter 2, where we'll delve into the fascinating world of macronutrients. These are the big players in your diet - carbohydrates, proteins, and fats. They provide the energy and building blocks your body needs for just about everything it does, from thinking to running marathons. Let's explore each of them in detail.

Carbohydrates: The Body's Preferred Fuel

Carbohydrates often get a bad rap in some trendy diets, but in reality, they are your body's preferred source of energy. Think of them as the gasoline in your car's tank - without enough carbs, you might sputter and stall.

Carbohydrates come in two main forms:

1. **Simple Carbohydrates:** These are the sugars, both natural (like those found in fruits and milk) and added sugars (like those in soda

and candy). They are quickly digested and provide a rapid energy boost, but they can also lead to energy crashes.

2. **Complex Carbohydrates:** These are starches and fibers found in foods like grains, legumes, and vegetables. They take longer to break down, providing a steady and sustained release of energy. Fiber, in particular, is crucial for digestive health and helps regulate blood sugar levels.

Carbs aren't just about energy, though. They play a vital role in brain function. Your brain relies almost entirely on glucose (a type of sugar) for fuel, and when glucose levels drop, you might experience difficulty concentrating and irritability - what many call "hanger."

Proteins: The Body's Builders

Proteins are often hailed as the body's building blocks, and with good reason. They are involved in just about every bodily function, from repairing tissues to producing enzymes and hormones. Every cell in your body contains proteins.

When you eat protein-rich foods like meat, fish, eggs, or plant sources like beans and tofu, your body breaks them down into amino acids. These amino acids are then used to build and repair tissues. Some amino acids are "essential," meaning your body can't make them, so you must get them from your diet.

Proteins aren't just about muscle, either. They play a role in immune function, producing energy when carbohydrates are scarce, and even in maintaining healthy hair and nails. So, when someone says "you are what you eat," remember that you're also made up of what you eat, and that's largely protein.

Fats: More Than Just Storage

Fats have long been demonized as the culprits behind weight gain and heart disease. However, fats are essential for your health, just like carbohydrates and proteins. They serve several vital functions in your body:

1. **Energy Storage:** Fats are highly concentrated sources of energy. They provide a backup source of fuel when carbohydrates are depleted.

2. **Cellular Structure:** Fats make up the lipid bilayer of your cell membranes, which controls what goes in and out of your cells. Without fats, your cells wouldn't function properly.

3. **Protection and Insulation:** Fats act as shock absorbers, protecting your vital organs. They also help insulate your body, keeping you warm in cold weather.

4. **Absorption of Fat-Soluble Vitamins:** Certain vitamins (A, D, E, and K) are fat-soluble, which means

they require dietary fat for absorption. Without fats, your body can't use these essential vitamins.

Now, not all fats are created equal. There are healthy fats and not-so-healthy fats:

- **Healthy Fats:** These include monounsaturated fats (found in olive oil, avocados, and nuts), polyunsaturated fats (found in fatty fish, flaxseeds, and walnuts), and some saturated fats (like those in coconut oil).

- **Not-So-Healthy Fats:** Trans fats (found in many processed and fried foods) and excessive saturated fats, especially from animal sources, can increase the risk of heart disease when consumed in large amounts.

So, when considering fats in your diet, think quality over quantity.

Balancing Macronutrients: The Key to a Healthy Diet

Balancing these macronutrients is key to a healthy diet. Different people have different needs based on their age, gender, activity level, and overall health. Here are some general guidelines:

- **Carbohydrates:** Aim to get most of your carbs from complex sources like whole grains, fruits, and vegetables. Limit added sugars and refined carbohydrates like white bread and sugary snacks.

- **Proteins:** Include a variety of protein sources in your diet. Lean meats, poultry, fish, eggs, dairy, legumes, and plant-based sources like tofu and tempeh are all excellent choices. Most people need more protein than they think, especially if they're physically active.

- **Fats:** Focus on unsaturated fats while minimizing saturated and trans fats. Include sources like avocados, nuts, seeds, and fatty fish in your diet. Remember that even healthy fats are calorie-dense, so moderation is key.

Special Diets and Macronutrients

Certain dietary choices, like vegetarianism and veganism, can impact your macronutrient intake.

Vegetarians avoid meat, while vegans exclude all animal products, including dairy and eggs.

If you're following one of these diets, it's crucial to plan your meals carefully to ensure you're getting all the essential nutrients. For example, plant-based diets might require extra attention to protein intake and vitamin B12 supplementation.

On the flip side, some diets, like low-carb or ketogenic diets, intentionally manipulate macronutrient ratios. These diets emphasize high-fat and low-carb intake, often with moderate protein. They aim to shift the body into a state of ketosis, where it burns fat for fuel instead of carbohydrates. While these diets can be effective for weight loss and managing certain medical conditions, they may not be suitable for everyone.

Beyond Macronutrients: The Role of Whole Foods

While macronutrients are essential, it's equally important to consider the source of these nutrients. Whole foods, as opposed to processed foods, provide a broader spectrum of nutrients, including vitamins, minerals, and fiber. They also tend to be more satiating, helping you manage your overall calorie intake.

Incorporating a variety of whole foods into your diet ensures that you're not only meeting your macronutrient needs but also supporting your overall health. It's like painting with a full palette of colors instead of just a few.

In summary, Chapter 2 has taken us on a journey through the world of macronutrients: carbohydrates, proteins, and fats. We've learned that each of these macronutrients plays a unique and vital role in our bodies, from providing energy to building and repairing tissues. We've also discussed the importance of balancing these macronutrients in our diet to support overall health.

Remember that no single macronutrient is "good" or "bad." It's about making informed choices and finding the right balance that suits your individual needs and goals. Whether you're an athlete looking to optimize performance or simply someone trying to maintain good health, understanding macronutrients is a

fundamental   step   toward
achieving your dietary objectives.

CHAPTER 3

Micronutrients - Vitamins and Minerals

Welcome to Chapter 3, where we'll embark on a journey into the world of micronutrients. These are the unsung heroes of your diet, often overlooked but essential for your health. We'll explore vitamins and minerals, understanding their roles, sources, and why they are crucial for your well-being.

Vitamins: Tiny but Mighty

Vitamins are organic compounds required in small amounts for various metabolic processes in your body. They play a vital role in maintaining good health and preventing diseases. Unlike macronutrients (carbohydrates, proteins, and fats), your body doesn't produce most vitamins, so you need to obtain them through your diet.

Let's delve into some of the key vitamins and their functions:

1. **Vitamin A:** Known for its role in maintaining healthy vision, vitamin A also supports your immune

system, skin, and the proper functioning of your heart, lungs, and kidneys. It can be found in foods like carrots, sweet potatoes, spinach, and dairy products.

2. **Vitamin C:** Often associated with citrus fruits, vitamin C is a powerful antioxidant that helps protect your cells from damage. It also aids in collagen production, which is essential for healthy skin, gums, and blood vessels.

3. **Vitamin D:** Sometimes referred to as the "sunshine vitamin" because your skin

can produce it when exposed to sunlight. Vitamin D is critical for calcium absorption, making it essential for strong bones and teeth.

4. **Vitamin E:** Another antioxidant, vitamin E helps protect your cells from oxidative damage. It also supports your immune system and skin health. Nuts, seeds, and vegetable oils are good sources of vitamin E.

5. **Vitamin K:** This vitamin is essential for blood clotting and bone health. Leafy

greens like spinach and kale, as well as broccoli, are rich in vitamin K.

6. **B Vitamins:** This group includes several vitamins, such as B1 (thiamine), B2 (riboflavin), B3 (niacin), B6 (pyridoxine), B9 (folate), and B12 (cobalamin). B vitamins are involved in energy metabolism, nerve function, and the production of red blood cells. They are found in a wide range of foods, including whole grains, meats, dairy products, and leafy greens.

7. **Vitamin B12:** This vitamin is unique because it's primarily found in animal products like meat, fish, and dairy. It's essential for nerve function and the production of DNA and RNA.

Minerals: The Building Blocks of Life

Minerals are inorganic substances that your body needs in relatively small quantities but are just as critical as vitamins for maintaining health. They serve various functions, including bone health, fluid balance, and nerve function. Here are some important minerals:

1. **Calcium:** Vital for strong bones and teeth, calcium is also involved in muscle function and blood clotting. Dairy products, leafy greens, and fortified foods are good sources.

2. **Iron:** Iron is a key component of hemoglobin, the protein in your red blood cells that carries oxygen to your body's tissues. Red meat, poultry, beans, and fortified cereals are iron-rich foods.

3. **Potassium:** This mineral helps regulate blood pressure, balance fluids, and support proper muscle and nerve function. Bananas, oranges, potatoes, and leafy greens are potassium-rich foods.

4. **Magnesium:** Magnesium is involved in hundreds of biochemical reactions in your body. It plays a role in muscle and nerve function, blood glucose control, and bone health. Nuts, seeds, whole grains, and leafy greens are good sources.

5. **Sodium:** While sodium is essential for fluid balance and nerve function, many people consume too much of it, often from processed foods. Reducing sodium intake is a focus for heart health.

6. **Zinc:** Zinc is essential for immune function, wound healing, and DNA synthesis. It can be found in meat, nuts, and whole grains.

7. **Selenium:** This mineral acts as an antioxidant and is essential for thyroid function. It's present in

foods like seafood, Brazil nuts, and poultry.

Deficiency and Toxicity: Striking the Right Balance

Getting the right amount of vitamins and minerals is crucial. Too little of a particular nutrient can lead to a deficiency, which can cause various health problems. Conversely, excessive intake can result in toxicity, which can also be harmful.

For example, a deficiency in vitamin C can lead to scurvy, which causes fatigue, muscle weakness, and bleeding gums. On the other hand, excessive intake of vitamin A can lead to toxicity symptoms like nausea, dizziness, and even hair loss.

That's why it's important to aim for a balanced diet that provides you with an adequate but not excessive amount of vitamins and minerals. Whole foods are an excellent way to achieve this balance because they often contain a variety of these nutrients in the right proportions.

The Case for Variety: Why Whole Foods Matter

Whole foods, such as fruits, vegetables, whole grains, lean proteins, and dairy products, offer a rich tapestry of vitamins and minerals. Consuming a wide variety of these foods ensures you receive a broad spectrum of nutrients, which can help prevent deficiencies and support overall health.

For example, an orange provides vitamin C, but it also contains small amounts of other vitamins and minerals like potassium and vitamin A. By eating a variety of foods, you can create a nutritional symphony that supports your well-being.

Conversely, highly processed foods are often stripped of many vitamins and minerals during manufacturing. They may be fortified with a few nutrients, but they rarely compare to the nutrient richness of whole foods. So, if you're looking to maximize your vitamin and mineral intake, focus on real, whole foods.

Bioavailability: Unlocking Nutrient Potential

Not all vitamins and minerals are created equal when it comes to how well your body can absorb and use them. Bioavailability refers to the extent and rate at which a nutrient is absorbed and used by the body.

Some factors affect bioavailability:

- **Nutrient Interactions:** Some nutrients enhance or inhibit the absorption of others. For instance, vitamin C can enhance the absorption of non-heme iron (the type of iron found in plant foods), so eating foods rich in vitamin C with iron-containing foods can boost iron absorption.

- **Food Preparation:** Cooking, processing, and even how you prepare foods can affect nutrient bioavailability. For instance, cooking tomatoes releases more lycopene, a potent antioxidant, making it more available for absorption.

- **Individual Factors:** Your individual health and genetics can also influence nutrient absorption. For example, some people have difficulty absorbing certain vitamins or minerals due to digestive conditions or genetic factors.

Supplements: A Double-Edged Sword

In some cases, dietary supplements can be beneficial, especially for individuals with specific deficiencies or those who have trouble meeting their nutritional needs through food alone. However, supplements should not be seen as a replacement for a balanced diet.

There are a few reasons for this:

1. **Synergy:** Nutrients often work together in a synergistic manner. They enhance each other's

absorption and effectiveness when obtained from whole foods. Isolating one nutrient in supplement form may not provide the same benefits.

2. **Unknowns:** The long-term effects of high-dose supplements aren't always clear, and some may even be harmful. For example, excessive vitamin E supplementation has been associated with an increased risk of bleeding.

3. **Absence of Other Nutrients:** Supplements can't replicate the complex mix of vitamins, minerals,

fiber, and other compounds found in whole foods. For example, an orange doesn't just provide vitamin C; it also offers fiber, antioxidants, and other health-promoting compounds.

In summary, Chapter 3 has been a deep dive into the world of micronutrients - vitamins and minerals. These tiny but mighty substances play critical roles in your health, from supporting your immune system to maintaining strong bones. We've explored various vitamins and minerals, their functions, sources, and the importance of getting the right balance. Remember that whole foods are your best bet for achieving this balance, as they offer a wide variety of nutrients in a bioavailable form. While supplements have their place, they should be used with caution and in consultation with a healthcare professional. By understanding and optimizing your intake of vitamins and minerals, you can take a significant step toward better health and well-being.

CHAPTER 4

Energy Balance and Weight Management

Welcome to Chapter 4, where we delve into the fascinating world of energy balance and weight management. This chapter is all about understanding the relationship between the calories you consume and the calories your body burns. It's a crucial concept for maintaining a healthy weight and overall well-being.

Energy Balance: The Fundamental Equation

At its core, weight management is a matter of energy balance - the equilibrium between the calories you consume through food and beverages and the calories your body expends for daily activities and metabolic processes. This balance dictates whether you gain, lose, or maintain weight.

The fundamental equation is quite simple:

- **Calories In (Consumed) - Calories Out (Burned) = Energy Balance**
- **Positive Energy Balance:** If you consistently consume more calories than your

body burns, you'll be in a positive energy balance. This leads to weight gain over time because the excess calories are stored as fat.

- **Negative Energy Balance:** On the other hand, if you consistently burn more calories than you consume, you'll be in a negative energy balance. This results in weight loss as your body taps into stored fat for energy.

- **Neutral Energy Balance:** When calories in and calories out are roughly equal, you'll maintain your current weight.

Understanding Your Basal Metabolic Rate (BMR)

A significant part of the energy your body burns daily goes into maintaining essential functions even at rest. This is known as your Basal Metabolic Rate (BMR). It includes functions like breathing, circulating blood, cell production, and tissue repair.

Several factors influence your BMR, including:

1. **Age:** BMR tends to decrease with age because lean

muscle mass typically decreases, and fat mass increases.

2. **Gender:** Generally, men tend to have a higher BMR than women because they typically have more muscle mass.

3. **Body Composition:** Muscle burns more calories at rest than fat. So, individuals with more muscle mass tend to have a higher BMR.

4. **Genetics:** Genetics play a role in determining your metabolic rate to some extent.

5. **Hormones:** Hormones like thyroid hormones can affect your BMR. An underactive thyroid can slow down metabolism.

Knowing your BMR can be a helpful starting point for managing your weight. It gives you an idea of how many calories your body needs just to maintain basic functions. You can then adjust your calorie intake and activity level to achieve your weight goals.

Calories In: The Role of Diet

Let's explore the "Calories In" part of the energy balance equation -

your calorie intake through food and beverages. This is where your dietary choices come into play.

1. **Caloric Needs:** To maintain your current weight, you need to consume the same number of calories that your body expends (calories out). If you want to lose weight, you'll need to create a calorie deficit by consuming fewer calories than you burn.

2. **Balanced Diet:** While calorie quantity is important, the quality of your diet matters as well. A

balanced diet that includes a variety of foods provides essential nutrients (as we explored in Chapter 2 and 3) and supports overall health.

3. **Portion Control:** It's not just what you eat but also how much. Portion control can help you manage your calorie intake, even if you're eating healthy foods.

4. **Mindful Eating:** Being mindful of what you eat and savoring your meals can help prevent overeating and promote a healthy relationship with food.

5. **Hydration:** Sometimes thirst can be mistaken for hunger. Staying adequately hydrated can help you differentiate between the two.

6. **Meal Timing:** Some people find that spreading their meals throughout the day and not skipping breakfast helps control hunger and manage calorie intake.

7. **Nutrient Density:** Opt for foods that are nutrient-dense, meaning they provide a lot of essential nutrients relative to their calorie content. Vegetables, fruits,

lean proteins, and whole grains are good examples.

Calories Out: The Role of Physical Activity

The "Calories Out" side of the equation involves the calories you burn through physical activity and daily life. It's not just about structured exercise but also the energy you expend during routine activities like walking, cleaning, or even fidgeting.

Here are some key points about the "Calories Out" side:

1. **Exercise:** Structured exercise, such as jogging,

swimming, or weightlifting, can significantly impact your calorie expenditure. The more vigorous the exercise, the more calories you'll burn during and after the workout.

2. **Non-Exercise Activity Thermogenesis (NEAT):** NEAT encompasses all the calories you burn during activities other than structured exercise. This includes walking, gardening, and even standing instead of sitting. Increasing NEAT can have a significant impact on your calorie expenditure.

3. **Basal Metabolic Rate (BMR):** As mentioned earlier, your BMR accounts for a significant portion of calories burned daily, even at rest.

4. **Thermic Effect of Food (TEF):** Your body expends calories to digest, absorb, and process the nutrients in the food you eat. This is known as the thermic effect of food. Protein-rich foods tend to have a higher TEF compared to fats and carbohydrates.

5. **Resting Metabolic Rate (RMR):** Similar to BMR,

RMR represents the number of calories your body burns at rest. It's influenced by factors like muscle mass and body composition.

6. **Individual Variation:** Everyone's calorie expenditure is different. Factors like genetics, age, and body composition play a role in determining how many calories you burn.

Strategies for Weight Management

Now that we understand the basics of energy balance, let's explore strategies for weight management:

1. **Calorie Tracking:** Keeping a food diary or using a calorie tracking app can help you become more aware of your calorie intake and make adjustments as needed.

2. **Meal Planning:** Planning your meals and snacks in advance can help you make healthier choices and control portion sizes.

3. **Physical Activity:** Incorporating regular physical activity into your routine not only burns calories but also offers numerous health benefits.

Find activities you enjoy to make it sustainable.

4. **Behavioral Changes:** Identifying triggers for overeating or unhealthy food choices and developing strategies to address them can be effective in managing weight.

5. **Gradual Changes:** Making small, sustainable changes to your diet and activity level can be more effective in the long term than drastic, unsustainable changes.

6. **Seeking Support:** For some individuals, seeking support from a registered

dietitian, nutritionist, or therapist can be beneficial in achieving and maintaining a healthy weight.

Weight Loss Myths and Realities

It's important to dispel some common myths about weight loss:

1. **Myth: Rapid Weight Loss is Best:** Crash diets and extreme weight loss programs may result in quick initial results, but they're often unsustainable and can harm your health in the long run.

2. **Myth: Carbohydrates are the Enemy:** Carbohydrates are an essential part of a balanced diet. It's the type and quantity of carbs that matter. Focus on whole grains and limit added sugars.

3. **Myth: Skipping Meals Helps You Lose Weight:** Skipping meals can lead to overeating later in the day and can slow down your metabolism.

4. **Myth: Certain Foods Burn Fat:** There's no magical fat-burning food.

Weight loss comes down to a sustained calorie deficit.

5. **Myth: Weight Loss is Linear:** Weight loss can be uneven. Your body may plateau at times, and that's normal. The key is to stay consistent with healthy habits.

Maintaining a Healthy Weight: Beyond the Scale

While weight is an important measure of health, it's not the only one. Other factors, such as body composition, fitness level, and overall well-being, should also be considered.

- **Body Composition:** Aim to build and maintain muscle mass while reducing excess body fat. This can be achieved through a combination of a balanced diet and regular physical activity.

- **Fitness Level:** Regular exercise contributes to cardiovascular health, strength, and flexibility, regardless of whether it leads to weight loss.

- **Health Metrics:** Monitoring other health metrics like blood pressure, cholesterol levels, and blood sugar is essential for a complete picture of your health.

- **Emotional Well-being:** Developing a healthy relationship with food and body image is crucial for long-term well-being.

In conclusion, Chapter 4 has provided an in-depth exploration of energy balance and weight management. Understanding the balance between calories consumed and calories expended is key to achieving and maintaining a healthy weight. By making informed choices about your diet, staying active, and adopting sustainable lifestyle changes, you can manage your weight and promote overall well-being. Remember that health is not solely defined by the number on the scale but also by factors like body composition, fitness level, and emotional well-being.

CHAPTER 5

Special Diets and Dietary Patterns

Welcome to Chapter 5, where we'll embark on a journey through the diverse landscape of special diets and dietary patterns. This chapter explores various eating styles that go beyond the basics of macronutrients and micronutrients. We'll dive into popular diets like vegetarianism, veganism, Mediterranean, and more, understanding their principles, benefits, and potential considerations.

Dietary Patterns: More Than Just Food

Before delving into specific diets, it's essential to understand the concept of dietary patterns. A dietary pattern is the overall composition of foods and beverages in a diet. It's not just about individual nutrients or isolated foods but rather the combination of foods and their frequency of consumption.

Dietary patterns can have a significant impact on health. For example, the Mediterranean diet, characterized by a high intake of fruits, vegetables, whole grains, and olive oil, has been associated with a reduced risk of heart disease and other chronic conditions.

The dietary patterns we adopt are often influenced by cultural, social, economic, and environmental factors. These patterns can vary widely among individuals and communities.

Vegetarianism: A Plant-Centric Lifestyle

Vegetarianism is a dietary pattern that excludes meat but may include other animal-derived foods like dairy and eggs. It's a broad category with various subtypes:

1. **Lacto-Ovo Vegetarian:** Excludes meat, fish, and poultry but includes dairy and eggs.

2. **Lacto Vegetarian:** Excludes meat, fish, poultry, and eggs but includes dairy products.

3. **Ovo Vegetarian:** Excludes meat, fish, poultry, and dairy but includes eggs.

4. **Vegan:** Excludes all animal-derived foods, including meat, fish, poultry, dairy, eggs, and honey.

Vegetarian diets have gained popularity for several reasons:

- **Health Benefits:** Vegetarian diets are often associated with lower risks of heart disease, high blood pressure, type 2 diabetes, and certain cancers.

- **Environmental Impact:** Plant-based diets tend to have a lower environmental footprint compared to diets rich in animal products.

- **Ethical and Moral Beliefs:** Many vegetarians choose this lifestyle for ethical reasons, such as animal welfare and concerns about factory farming.

- **Cultural and Religious Traditions:** Some cultures and religions promote vegetarianism as a way of life.

To maintain a healthy vegetarian diet, it's essential to ensure you're getting adequate protein, vitamin B12, iron, calcium, and other nutrients typically found in animal-derived foods. Plant-based protein sources include beans, lentils, tofu, nuts, and seeds. Nutritional supplements may also be necessary, especially for vitamin B12.

Veganism: A Plant-Exclusive Lifestyle

Veganism takes vegetarianism a step further by excluding all animal-derived foods. It's a lifestyle choice that extends beyond diet to encompass a commitment to not using or supporting products derived from animals, including clothing and cosmetics.

While veganism offers health and environmental benefits similar to vegetarianism, it requires careful attention to nutrition to ensure you're meeting all your dietary needs:

- **Protein:** Plant-based sources like legumes, tofu, tempeh, and seitan can provide ample protein. Nuts and seeds are also good options.

- **Vitamin B12:** Since this vitamin is primarily found in animal products, vegans often need a B12 supplement or fortified foods.

- **Iron:** Plant-based sources of iron include fortified cereals, lentils, chickpeas, tofu, and dark leafy greens. Pairing iron-rich foods with vitamin C-rich foods can enhance absorption.

- **Calcium:** Fortified plant-based milk, tofu, and leafy greens like kale and collard greens are calcium sources.

- **Omega-3 Fatty Acids:** Flaxseeds, chia seeds, hemp

seeds, and walnuts are rich in alpha-linolenic acid (ALA), a type of omega-3 fatty acid. Consider algae-based supplements for longer-chain omega-3s like EPA and DHA.

Flexitarianism: A Flexible Approach

Flexitarianism, or the "flexible vegetarian" diet, is a dietary pattern that combines elements of vegetarianism with occasional consumption of meat or fish. It's a flexible approach that allows individuals to enjoy the health and environmental benefits of plant-based eating while still enjoying animal-derived foods in moderation.

The flexibility of this approach makes it more accessible to people who may not want to commit to a strict vegetarian or vegan lifestyle. It encourages a greater focus on plant-based foods while allowing room for personal preferences and occasional indulgences.

Paleo Diet: Eating Like Our Ancestors

The Paleolithic, or Paleo, diet aims to mimic the dietary patterns of our ancient ancestors, focusing on foods presumed to have been available to them during the Stone Age. It includes:

- Lean meats
- Fish
- Fruits
- Vegetables
- Nuts
- Seeds

The diet excludes:

- Grains
- Legumes
- Dairy
- Processed foods
- Sugars
- Alcohol

The rationale behind the Paleo diet is that our bodies are genetically adapted to the diet of our ancestors and that modern diets, especially those high in processed foods and grains, contribute to various health issues.

While the Paleo diet emphasizes whole foods and can lead to weight loss and improved blood sugar control, it's not without criticism. Some argue that it oversimplifies human evolution and doesn't consider the significant dietary variation among our ancient ancestors.

Ketogenic Diet: The Low-Carb, High-Fat Approach

The ketogenic diet, or keto diet, is a high-fat, low-carb eating plan designed to shift the body into a state of ketosis. Ketosis occurs when the body runs low on carbohydrates and starts using fat for fuel, producing ketones in the process.

The typical macronutrient breakdown of a keto diet is approximately:

- 70-75% fat
- 20-25% protein
- 5-10% carbohydrates

The diet emphasizes:

- Fatty cuts of meat
- Fish
- Eggs
- Full-fat dairy
- Avocado
- Nuts and seeds
- Oils like olive oil and coconut oil

The diet restricts:

- Grains
- Legumes
- Sugars
- Starchy vegetables

- Fruits (except for small portions of low-carb options)

The ketogenic diet has gained popularity for its potential benefits in weight loss, blood sugar control, and epilepsy treatment. However, it's not suitable for everyone and can have side effects like the "keto flu" during the initial adjustment period.

Mediterranean Diet: A Heart-Healthy Lifestyle

The Mediterranean diet is inspired by the traditional dietary patterns of countries bordering the

Mediterranean Sea, such as Greece, Italy, and Spain. It's renowned for its heart-healthy benefits and includes:

- Fruits and vegetables
- Whole grains
- Olive oil as the primary fat source
- Lean protein sources like fish, poultry, and legumes
- Nuts and seeds
- Moderate consumption of red wine (optional)
- Limited red meat and processed foods

The Mediterranean diet is rich in antioxidants, healthy fats, and fiber, making it effective in reducing the risk of heart disease, stroke, and certain cancers. It's also associated with improved cognitive function and longevity.

Intermittent Fasting: Timing Matters

Intermittent fasting isn't about what you eat but when you eat. It involves cycling between periods of eating and fasting. There are several popular methods:

1. **16/8 Method:** This involves fasting for 16 hours and eating during an 8-hour window.

2. **5:2 Diet:** In this approach, you consume your usual diet for five days and restrict calorie intake to around 500-600 calories on two non-consecutive days.

3. **Eat-Stop-Eat:** This method involves a 24-hour fast once or twice a week.

4. **Alternate-Day Fasting:** You alternate between days of normal eating and days of either fasting or very low-calorie intake.

Intermittent fasting may offer benefits like weight loss, improved insulin sensitivity, and potential longevity effects. However, it may not be suitable for everyone, and it's essential to consult a healthcare provider before starting any fasting regimen.

Considerations for Special Diets

While these dietary patterns offer various potential benefits, there are considerations to keep in mind:

- **Nutritional Adequacy:** Ensure you're meeting your nutrient needs, especially if you follow a restrictive diet. Consider consulting a

registered dietitian or
healthcare provider for
guidance.

- **Sustainability:** Choose a
dietary pattern that you can
maintain in the long term.
Diets that are too restrictive
or challenging to follow are
less likely to be sustainable.

- **Individual Variation:**
What works for one person
may not work for another.
Individual factors like
genetics, age, and health
conditions can influence
dietary needs and responses.

- **Balance:** Aim for a
balanced diet that includes a

variety of foods to ensure you're getting a wide range of nutrients.

In conclusion, Chapter 5 has explored special diets and dietary patterns that go beyond the basics of macronutrients and micronutrients. Whether you choose a vegetarian, vegan, flexitarian, Paleo, ketogenic, Mediterranean, or intermittent fasting approach, it's essential to understand the principles, benefits, and potential considerations of each dietary pattern. Remember that individual needs and preferences vary, so choose a dietary pattern that aligns with your goals and lifestyle while ensuring nutritional adequacy and balance.

CHAPTER 6

Nutrition Across the Lifespan

Welcome to Chapter 6, where we'll embark on a journey through the various stages of life and how nutrition plays a vital role in each. From infancy to old age, our nutritional needs evolve, and understanding these changes is essential for maintaining health and well-being throughout our lives.

Nutrition in Infancy: Building a Strong Foundation

The journey of nutrition begins at birth and even before. During pregnancy, a mother's diet plays a crucial role in the development of the fetus. Proper prenatal nutrition ensures the baby receives essential nutrients for growth and development.

Once born, breastfeeding is often recommended as the best source of nutrition for infants. Breast milk provides the perfect blend of nutrients, including proteins, fats, carbohydrates, vitamins, and minerals. It also contains antibodies that help protect against infections.

For infants who are not breastfed, infant formula is designed to mimic the nutritional composition of breast milk as closely as possible.

Key nutrients for infants include:

1. **Protein:** Essential for growth and tissue repair.

2. **Fats:** Provide energy and are crucial for brain development.

3. **Carbohydrates:** Serve as an energy source.

4. **Vitamins and Minerals:** Support various bodily functions.

5. **Iron:** Important for cognitive development and preventing anemia.

As infants grow, they transition to solid foods, typically starting with single-grain cereals and progressing to fruits, vegetables, lean proteins, and dairy products. The introduction of new foods should be gradual, and attention should be paid to potential allergens.

Childhood Nutrition: Fuel for Growth and Development

Childhood is a period of rapid growth and development, both physically and mentally. Proper nutrition during this stage is critical for:

1. **Growth:** Adequate intake of proteins, vitamins, and minerals supports physical growth.
2. **Cognitive Development:** Nutrients like omega-3 fatty

acids and iron are essential for brain development.

3. **Immune Function:** A balanced diet helps build a strong immune system.

4. **Establishing Healthy Habits:** Childhood is a crucial time to develop lifelong healthy eating habits.

It's important to encourage a varied diet that includes fruits, vegetables, whole grains, lean proteins, and dairy products. Avoid excessive intake of sugary and processed foods, which can contribute to weight gain and dental issues.

Adolescence: Nutritional Needs Amid Growth Spurts

Adolescence is marked by rapid growth, hormonal changes, and increased physical activity. Proper nutrition during this phase is essential for:

1. **Growth and Development:** Adolescents are still growing, and they require nutrients for bone development, muscle growth, and hormonal changes.

2. **Energy Needs:** Increased physical activity means higher energy requirements.

3. **Iron Needs:** Especially important for girls due to the onset of menstruation.

4. **Calcium:** Important for bone health.

However, this is also a time when dietary habits can shift towards less healthy choices, like fast food and sugary drinks. Parents and caregivers play a crucial role in guiding adolescents toward balanced eating habits.

Nutrition in Adulthood: Maintaining Health and Preventing Disease

Adulthood is a stage where maintaining health and preventing disease become priorities. Key considerations include:

1. **Energy Balance:** As metabolism tends to slow with age, managing calorie intake and staying physically active become increasingly important to prevent weight gain.

2. **Bone Health:** Adequate calcium and vitamin D intake are crucial for

maintaining bone density, especially for women approaching menopause.

3. **Heart Health:** A heart-healthy diet low in saturated and trans fats can help prevent cardiovascular disease.

4. **Cancer Prevention:** Certain dietary patterns, like those rich in fruits, vegetables, and whole grains, are associated with a reduced risk of cancer.

5. **Fiber Intake:** Fiber helps with digestion and can lower the risk of chronic diseases like diabetes.

6. **Hydration:** Staying well-hydrated becomes more critical as the sensation of thirst may diminish with age.

It's important to adopt a balanced diet that includes a variety of nutrient-dense foods and to stay physically active. Regular check-ups with healthcare providers can help identify and address nutritional concerns or health issues.

Nutrition During Pregnancy and Lactation: Supporting Two Lives

Pregnancy is a unique time in a woman's life when her nutritional needs increase to support both her own health and the developing fetus. Key nutrients during pregnancy include:

1. **Folic Acid:** Important for early neural tube development.
2. **Iron:** Necessary for the increased blood volume and oxygen transport to the fetus.
3. **Calcium and Vitamin D:** Essential for the development of the baby's bones and teeth.

4. **Omega-3 Fatty Acids:** Support fetal brain and eye development.

5. **Protein:** Required for the growth of the placenta and the baby.

During lactation, the mother's diet continues to be crucial as it affects the composition of breast milk. Adequate calorie intake, hydration, and a balanced diet remain important to ensure both mother and baby receive the necessary nutrients.

Breast milk is considered the gold standard for infant nutrition, providing essential nutrients and immune-boosting factors. However, for various reasons, some mothers may need to supplement with formula.

Nutrition in Older Adults: Nourishing Aging Bodies

As individuals age, their nutritional needs may change due to factors like decreased metabolism, changes in body composition, and potential health conditions. Key considerations for nutrition in older adults include:

1. **Caloric Needs:** Energy requirements may decrease, making portion control

important to prevent weight gain.

2. **Protein:** Adequate protein intake is essential for preserving muscle mass.

3. **Calcium and Vitamin D:** Important for bone health.

4. **Fiber:** Helps with digestion and may help lower the risk of constipation.

5. **Hydration:** Older adults may be at a higher risk of dehydration.

6. **Vitamin B12:** Absorption of this vitamin can decrease with age, so B12 supplements or fortified foods may be necessary.

7. **Sodium:** Reducing sodium intake can help manage blood pressure, which is important for cardiovascular health.

Special Considerations in Older Adults:

- **Malnutrition:** Older adults are at risk of malnutrition due to factors like reduced appetite, dental problems, and limited mobility.

- **Chronic Conditions:** Certain medical conditions like diabetes or heart disease may require specific dietary modifications.

- **Medication Interactions:** Some medications can affect nutrient absorption or metabolism, so it's essential to discuss these with healthcare providers.

- **Social Isolation:** Loneliness or living alone can impact eating habits and nutrition, making social support crucial.

In conclusion, Chapter 6 has explored nutrition across the lifespan, emphasizing the importance of tailoring dietary choices to meet the unique needs of each life stage. From infancy to old age, proper nutrition plays a fundamental role in growth, development, and overall health. Understanding these nutritional needs and making informed choices is key to promoting well-being throughout life. Additionally, it's important to consider factors like cultural preferences, lifestyle, and individual health status when planning and implementing a healthy diet at any age.

CHAPTER 7

Nutritional Challenges and Controversies

Welcome to Chapter 7, where we delve into the complex and often contentious world of nutritional challenges and controversies. Nutrition is a field rife with debates, evolving science, and diverse opinions. This chapter explores some of the most significant challenges and controversies in nutrition, providing insights into the factors that contribute to these debates and offering evidence-based perspectives.

1. Fad Diets: The Allure and Risks

Fad diets are diets that gain sudden popularity, promising rapid weight loss or other health benefits. They often rely on extreme restrictions, unusual food combinations, or specific food groups, leading to rapid initial weight loss. However, the long-term success and safety of these diets are often questionable.

Examples of fad diets include:

- **Keto Diet:** A high-fat, low-carbohydrate diet designed to induce ketosis, a state where the body burns fat for fuel.

- **Detox or Cleanse Diets:** These diets claim to rid the body of toxins but often involve severe calorie restriction and the elimination of entire food groups.

- **Juice Cleanses:** Replacing meals with fruit or vegetable juices for a set period, which can lead to nutrient deficiencies.

The allure of fad diets lies in their promises of quick results. However, they often lack scientific support, can be nutritionally unbalanced, and may not be sustainable in the long run. Many people find that the weight lost on fad diets is often regained once normal eating patterns resume.

A balanced, sustainable diet that includes a variety of nutrient-dense foods remains the most reliable approach to long-term health and weight management.

2. Conflicting Dietary Guidelines

Nutritional guidelines are recommendations issued by government agencies or health organizations to help the public make informed dietary choices. However, there can be conflicts or contradictions between different sets of guidelines, leading to confusion for consumers.

For instance, debates around dietary fat have been ongoing. In the past, low-fat diets were widely recommended to reduce the risk of heart disease. However, more recent guidelines have shifted towards a focus on the type of fats consumed rather than simply reducing overall fat intake. Healthy fats, like those found in avocados and nuts, are now promoted as part of a balanced diet.

The best approach for individuals is to consult guidelines from reputable sources, such as the Dietary Guidelines for Americans or the World Health Organization, and to consider individual health conditions, preferences, and cultural factors.

3. Sugar: The Sweet Controversy

Sugar has become a central point of controversy in nutrition. Excessive sugar consumption has been linked to obesity, type 2 diabetes, heart disease, and dental problems. The debate centers on whether added sugars are more harmful than naturally occurring sugars found in whole foods like fruits and dairy.

- **Added Sugars:** These are sugars added to foods during processing, often to improve flavor. They include ingredients like sucrose, high-fructose corn syrup, and various syrups and sweeteners.

- **Naturally Occurring Sugars:** These sugars are found naturally in foods like fruits (fructose) and dairy products (lactose).

Current dietary guidelines often recommend limiting added sugars but not naturally occurring sugars, as the latter come with essential nutrients and fiber. However, it's essential to consider the overall context of one's diet.

The controversy also extends to sugar substitutes or artificial sweeteners. While they are marketed as low-calorie alternatives, some studies suggest that they may not necessarily lead to weight loss and may have their own set of potential health concerns.

In navigating the sugar controversy, it's wise to limit added sugars and focus on whole, minimally processed foods while still enjoying naturally occurring sugars in moderation.

4. Organic vs. Conventional Foods

The choice between organic and conventional foods has sparked significant debate. Organic foods are produced without synthetic pesticides, herbicides, or genetically modified organisms (GMOs), while conventional foods may use these practices.

Proponents of organic foods argue that they are more environmentally friendly and may contain fewer pesticide residues. Some also claim that organic foods are more nutritious, although the scientific consensus on this is still evolving.

Conversely, critics argue that organic foods are more expensive and not significantly more nutritious than conventional foods. They also point out that some synthetic pesticides used in conventional farming have been extensively tested for safety.

The choice between organic and conventional foods often comes down to personal values, budget constraints, and individual health concerns. Washing fruits and vegetables thoroughly can help reduce pesticide residues on conventional produce, while opting for organic foods may align with environmental or ethical considerations.

5. Genetically Modified Organisms (GMOs)

Genetically modified organisms, or GMOs, are organisms whose genetic material has been altered in a way that does not occur naturally. In agriculture, GMOs are often engineered to resist pests, diseases, or herbicides, or to enhance crop yield.

The controversy surrounding GMOs centers on concerns about their safety for human consumption and potential environmental impacts. Advocates argue that GMOs have the potential to increase crop yields, reduce pesticide use, and enhance nutrient content. However, critics express concerns about the long-term health effects and unintended consequences of GMOs.

The scientific consensus, supported by organizations like the World Health Organization and the National Academy of Sciences, is that GMOs currently approved for consumption are safe to eat. However, ongoing research and rigorous testing are essential to ensure safety.

6. Nutritional Supplements: Bridging the Gap or Risking Harm?

Nutritional supplements, including vitamins, minerals, and herbal products, have gained popularity as a way to fill nutrient gaps in one's diet or address specific health concerns.

The controversy surrounding supplements revolves around their necessity and safety. While supplements can be beneficial for individuals with specific nutrient deficiencies or medical conditions, they are not a substitute for a balanced diet.

Some concerns related to supplements include:

- **Safety:** Quality control can vary among supplement manufacturers, leading to potential risks of contamination or incorrect labeling.

- **Effectiveness:** Not all supplements have been proven effective in scientific studies.

- **Interaction with Medications:** Some supplements can interact with medications, potentially causing harmful effects.

- **Overconsumption:**
  Excessive intake of certain vitamins and minerals can be harmful.

It's advisable to consult with a healthcare provider before taking supplements to assess individual needs and potential risks. In most cases, obtaining nutrients from whole foods is the safest and most effective approach.

7. Nutritional Confusion in the Age of Information

The digital age has brought a wealth of information on nutrition to our fingertips. While this can be empowering, it has also led to confusion due to the abundance of conflicting advice, sensationalized headlines, and misinformation.

Several factors contribute to nutritional confusion:

- **Media Hype:** Headlines promoting "superfoods" or "miracle diets" can distort the perception of what constitutes a healthy diet.

- **Sensationalism:** Misleading or exaggerated health claims can spread quickly on social media, leading to unfounded dietary trends.

- **Individualization:** Nutrition is highly individualized, and what works for one person may not work for another, leading to conflicting anecdotes.

- **Cherry-Picking Data:** Studies with intriguing findings can be overemphasized, even if they don't represent the overall scientific consensus.

Navigating the sea of nutritional information requires critical thinking, an understanding of the scientific method, and reliance on reputable sources like government health agencies, academic institutions, and registered dietitians.

In conclusion, Chapter 7 has explored some of the most significant nutritional challenges and controversies that exist in the field of nutrition. From fad diets to conflicting dietary guidelines, debates over sugar, organic vs. conventional foods, GMOs, and the use of nutritional supplements, the world of nutrition is complex and ever-evolving. In the age of information, it's crucial to approach these controversies with a critical eye, rely on evidence-based guidance, and consider individual health needs and values when making dietary choices. Ultimately, a balanced and diverse diet, rich in whole, minimally processed foods, remains a solid foundation for good nutrition.

CHAPTER 8

The Future of Nutrition and Diet Therapy

Welcome to the final chapter, where we explore the exciting frontier of the future of nutrition and diet therapy. As our understanding of nutrition advances and technology evolves, this field is poised for significant innovations and transformations. In this chapter, we'll delve into some key areas where the future of nutrition and diet therapy is taking shape.

1. Personalized Nutrition: Tailoring Diets to Individuals

One of the most promising developments in nutrition is the move towards personalized nutrition. Rather than adhering to one-size-fits-all dietary recommendations, the future of nutrition will increasingly consider individual factors like genetics, metabolism, gut microbiome composition, and even personal preferences and goals.

Genetic Testing: Genetic testing can reveal how your genes may influence your response to different foods and nutrients. For example, some people may have a genetic predisposition that makes them more responsive to a low-carb diet, while others may thrive on a balanced diet with moderate carbohydrate intake.

Microbiome Analysis: Research on the gut microbiome, the community of microorganisms living in your digestive tract, is unveiling how it impacts digestion, metabolism, and overall health. Future diets may be customized based on an individual's unique microbiome composition.

Metabolic Profiling: Advanced metabolic profiling can provide insights into how your body processes different nutrients. This information can help tailor dietary recommendations to optimize energy balance and weight management.

Artificial Intelligence: AI-powered algorithms can analyze vast amounts of data to generate personalized dietary recommendations. Apps and devices may use AI to track your diet, monitor your health, and offer real-time guidance.

2. Nutrigenomics: The Gene-Nutrient Connection

Nutrigenomics is the study of how genes interact with nutrients and how diet can influence gene expression. This emerging field holds the potential to revolutionize nutrition therapy by uncovering how specific dietary patterns can be used to prevent or treat genetic-based health conditions.

For example, researchers are exploring how dietary interventions can modulate gene expression to reduce the risk of conditions like heart disease, diabetes, and cancer. Nutrigenomic insights may lead to highly targeted dietary recommendations that help individuals optimize their health based on their genetic profile.

3. Functional Foods and Nutraceuticals

Functional foods are foods with added health benefits beyond basic nutrition. Nutraceuticals, on the other hand, are dietary supplements that may have medicinal properties. These categories encompass a wide range of products, from probiotic-enriched yogurt to antioxidant-rich teas.

The future of nutrition will likely see an expansion of functional foods and nutraceuticals designed to address specific health concerns. These products may target conditions such as inflammation, cognitive decline, or bone health. However, it's crucial that these claims are supported by robust scientific evidence and regulatory oversight to ensure their safety and efficacy.

4. The Role of Technology

Technology will continue to play a significant role in shaping the future of nutrition and diet therapy. Here are some ways technology is transforming this field:

Wearable Devices: Wearable fitness and health trackers can monitor your physical activity, heart rate, and even sleep patterns. These devices can provide valuable data for dietitians and healthcare providers when creating personalized nutrition plans.

Mobile Apps: Nutrition apps can help users track their food intake, provide nutritional information, and offer personalized meal plans. These apps can also connect users with dietitians and provide real-time feedback and guidance.

Telehealth and Virtual Care: Telehealth services allow individuals to consult with healthcare professionals, including dietitians, remotely. This technology makes it easier for people to access expert dietary guidance, regardless of their location.

Nutrition Genomics Platforms: Online platforms that combine genetic data with nutritional insights are emerging. These platforms provide users with personalized dietary recommendations based on their genetic profile.

5. Sustainable Eating: Considerations Beyond Health

As concerns about climate change and environmental sustainability continue to grow, the future of nutrition will place greater emphasis on sustainable eating. This means considering the environmental impact of food choices in addition to health factors.

Plant-Based Diets: Plant-based diets, such as vegetarianism and veganism, are not only associated with health benefits but also have a lower environmental footprint compared to diets rich in animal products.

Locally Sourced Foods: Supporting local and regional food systems can reduce the carbon footprint associated with transporting food long distances.

Reducing Food Waste: Strategies to reduce food waste, such as meal planning and proper storage, can contribute to sustainability efforts.

Sustainable Farming Practices: Encouraging sustainable farming practices that reduce chemical use and promote soil health can benefit both human health and the environment.

6. Global Nutrition Challenges

The future of nutrition and diet therapy will continue to grapple with global nutrition challenges, including:

Malnutrition: Despite advances in nutrition science, malnutrition remains a critical issue, affecting both undernourished and overnourished populations. Innovative strategies are needed to address these complex challenges.

Food Security: Ensuring that everyone has access to safe, nutritious, and culturally appropriate food is a global priority. Addressing food security requires a combination of policies, education, and sustainable agricultural practices.

Nutrition Education: Nutrition education will play a vital role in improving public health. Teaching individuals how to make informed dietary choices is essential for preventing diet-related diseases.

Addressing Health Disparities: Reducing health disparities related to nutrition is a crucial goal. Ensuring that marginalized communities have access to affordable, healthy food options is essential.

In conclusion, the future of nutrition and diet therapy holds exciting possibilities, from personalized nutrition and nutrigenomics to functional foods, technology integration, and sustainable eating. These developments have the potential to transform the way we approach nutrition and lead to more effective dietary interventions that enhance both individual and public health. However, it's essential that these advancements are guided by rigorous scientific research and a commitment to addressing global nutrition challenges to ensure a healthier and more sustainable future for all.

CONCLUSION

In conclusion, the journey through the eight chapters on nutrition and diet therapy has provided a comprehensive exploration of this multifaceted field. Here, we summarize the key takeaways from each chapter and tie them together into a cohesive conclusion.

Chapter 1: Foundations of Nutrition

- Nutrition is the science of how the body uses nutrients

from food for growth, maintenance, and health.

- Nutrients can be categorized into macronutrients (carbohydrates, proteins, fats) and micronutrients (vitamins and minerals).
- A balanced diet that includes a variety of foods is crucial for meeting nutrient needs.

Chapter 2: Digestion, Absorption, and Metabolism

- The digestive system breaks down food into nutrients that can be absorbed into the bloodstream.

- Enzymes and hormones play key roles in digestion and nutrient absorption.

- Metabolism is the body's process of using nutrients for energy and other functions.

Chapter 3: Nutrient Requirements and Dietary Reference Intakes

- Nutrient requirements vary based on age, gender, activity level, and life stage.

- Dietary Reference Intakes (DRIs) provide guidelines for nutrient intake to meet health needs.

- DRIs include Recommended Dietary Allowances (RDAs), Adequate Intakes (AIs), Tolerable Upper Intake Levels (ULs), and Estimated Average Requirements (EARs).

Chapter 4: Energy Balance and Weight Management

- Energy balance is the relationship between calorie intake and expenditure.
- To lose weight, you must create a calorie deficit; to gain weight, a surplus is needed.

- Weight management goes beyond the scale and includes factors like body composition and overall well-being.

Chapter 5: Special Diets and Dietary Patterns

- Vegetarian, vegan, flexitarian, Paleo, ketogenic, Mediterranean, and intermittent fasting diets are popular dietary patterns.
- Each dietary pattern has its principles, benefits, and considerations.
- Individualization is crucial in choosing a dietary pattern

that aligns with health goals and lifestyle.

Chapter 6: Nutrition Across the Lifespan

- Nutritional needs evolve throughout life, from infancy to old age.

- Proper nutrition is critical for growth, development, and overall health at every stage.

- Factors like genetics, lifestyle, and cultural preferences influence dietary choices.

Chapter 7: Nutritional Challenges and Controversies

- Fad diets, conflicting dietary guidelines, sugar controversies, organic vs. conventional foods, GMOs, and nutritional supplements are sources of debate in nutrition.

- Critical thinking and reliance on reputable sources are essential for navigating nutritional controversies.

- Nutrition misinformation can be prevalent in the

digital age, requiring a discerning approach.

Chapter 8: The Future of Nutrition and Diet Therapy

- The future of nutrition is marked by personalized nutrition, nutrigenomics, functional foods, technology integration, sustainable eating, and addressing global nutrition challenges.
- Personalized nutrition considers individual factors like genetics, microbiome, and metabolism.
- Sustainability and technology will play

significant roles in shaping the future of nutrition.

In summary, nutrition and diet therapy are dynamic and ever-evolving fields that impact every aspect of our lives. Proper nutrition is fundamental for health and well-being, and understanding the science of nutrition empowers individuals to make informed dietary choices. As the future unfolds, personalized nutrition, technological advancements, and sustainable practices promise to further enhance our ability to optimize health and address global nutrition challenges. However, it's essential to approach these developments with a critical and evidence-based mindset to ensure a healthier and more nourished world for all.